Dr.Purissima M.Glaze

BEAUTY IS HEALTH MADE VISIBLE

(SELF EVIDENT OF HEALTHY BEAUTY)

Dr.Purissima M.Glaze

Copyright © 2022 by Dr.Purissima M.Glaze

All rights reserved.

Dr.Purissima M.Glaze

INTRODUCTION

These days we are showing more worry for beauty than for health. This propensity is perhaps impacted by a few variables - social cycles, job of promotions and broad communications, neighborhood and worldwide patterns in the design business, and reception of unfamiliar social practices. This article gives a scrutinize of the fixation for beauty, contends for additional investigation into this peculiarity and requires the improvement of health advancement projects to enhance this pattern.

Chapter 1

3 Different ways Beauty Can Effect Your Health and Prosperity

In any case, what does indeed "healthy beauty" mean?

SELF is a health brand, and that implies that we approach all that we make and distribute from the perspective of health. As the senior beauty proofreader, I'm continuously contemplating how to cover my beat such that will serve our focal mission of assisting individuals with feeling improved. Our image theory is that feeling good in your skin is as crucial for living great as eating supporting food varieties, getting sufficient rest, or moving your body; in that sense, beauty (and all it involves) in inseparably attached to health.

However, what does "healthy beauty" mean, as a matter of fact? With our healthy beauty bundle, we're celebrating three unmistakable mainstays of it: dealing with yourself, being an educated customer, and articulating your thoughts. This is the way we're tending to every one of those points of support.

Dr.Purissima M.Glaze

1. Dealing with yourself

Health conditions that influence the manner in which you look can have a profound effect, and figuring out how to live with and deal with those health conditions and their side effects can be a significant road toward feeling improved truly and mentally. Past the more clinical applications, beauty items and schedules can likewise be devices for taking care of oneself overall — I'm talking shower bombs and facial coverings for unwinding, obviously, albeit the demonstration of dealing with yourself goes a lot further than that.

We want to be an asset of precise and master endorsed item suggestions, counsel, and intel for all that from skin disease to dandruff, and we work intimately with dermatologists, restorative scientific experts, and researchers to present to you the most exceptional, research-supported data. Simultaneously, we likewise include stories from individuals living with those conditions consistently, sharing their own interpretation of how beauty assists them with feeling quite a bit improved.

2. Being an educated shopper

Beauty paths are flooded with items showcased as "clean" and "regular." Yet how do you have at least some idea which fixings are truly worth stressing over? We take a gander at the science behind the cases to assist you with better grasping what's genuine, what's publicity, and what we do and don't really have any idea.

All things considered, we as a whole are about private decision with regards to what you put on or in your body. There are a ton of lab-made fixings out there that are really viable and safe, however in the event that you like to go normal with your beauty standard, that is a substantial individual choice. We want to assist you with settling on the best decisions for yourself by furnishing you with the most ideal data that anyone could hope to find — which incorporates ensuring you know that "normal" doesn't have a severe definition with regards to beauty care products, and that it's not inseparable from "safe" or "delicate." That is the reason everything except one of the classes of grants this year don't zero in on "regular" items by any means. (The one classification that does — The 11 Best Regular Skin-Care and Cosmetics Items is for those of you who are still about that normal beauty life, since we got you covered.) In the mean time, read "What the Exploration Says Regarding 10 Questionable Beauty care products Fixings" to get the overview on those terrifying sounding fixings everybody continues to discuss, and ideally feel a piece less blew a gasket and confounded.

3. Articulating your thoughts

Beauty items can be striking and enchanted instruments that assist you with communicating your own personality and style, upgrade what makes you one of a kind, and feel your best. The manner in which you do — or don't do — your hair and cosmetics is one method for assisting you with feeling most such as yourself. Furthermore, as beauty organizations center more around inclusivity by offering a more extensive scope of items, more individuals will actually want to approach those devices that assist them with feeling most at ease in their own skin.

So whether you have straight hair, unusual hair, earthy colored skin, or spots, we need to share data and stories that impact you, and address your look and way of life.

At SELF, healthy beauty is private, and we're continuously finding out more.

Dr.Purissima M.Glaze

Chapter 2

Assuming Beauty Is Health Made Apparent, What Does Your Skin Say Regarding You?

Lively SKINCARE

beauty, lively skincare, skincare

Health and beauty require stream and equilibrium of fundamental energy all through the body. Stylish issues frequently are indications of enthusiastic lopsidedness, or something 'messed up. In the event that this sounds accurate for yourself and beauty is, truth be told, health made noticeable - what is your skin talking about your health?

Keeping up with and reestablishing vigorous equilibrium is at the center of beauty and health (physical, profound, and mental) and your skin is an immediate impression of internal operations.

Think: Dry or slick skin, skin break out, scars, amplified pores, fine kinks, or puffy eyes. With regards to your body, think: cellulite, dry skin, bug veins, puffiness, and stretch imprints. These actual signs are a consequence of inward lopsidedness.

With everything that expressed, how might you better deal with your health and consider it your skin?

Reflect - Contemplation can be polished in various ways. In spite of the fact that it is a customary discipline for the majority profoundly spurred individuals, it can likewise be utilized in pressure the board, unwinding and by and large, in many types of self-mending. As per our companions at Phytobiodermie, numerous ever-evolving medical clinics show their patients some reflective practice since they have recorded the connected physical and close to home advantages. Assuming it is great for your health, it is great for your skin!

Pick the Right Skin Care Items - Phytobiodermie is a trailblazer in seepage (with the Boidraineur) presently viewed as a pre-essential for a quality facial or body treatment. Phytobiodermie additionally presented the utilization of Light-Treatment (with the Chromapuncteur). It opens vast opportunities for prepared specialists as light-treatment is an effortless and harmless methodology with results like needle therapy.

Work out - Obviously practice is perfect for your heart, lungs, and mental viewpoint. In any case, here's one more motivation to get going: Customary activity is one of the keys to healthy skin. By expanding blood stream, practice feeds skin cells and keep them indispensable

Spoil Yourself Occasionally - Come by and see us for a select skin care treatment. Weiler Foundation is currently adjusting the brain and body through vivacious skincare. This most recent contribution is an interesting and critical part to accomplishing and keeping up with all encompassing health. This creative and compelling skincare program works with the energy of the body to mend, recover, and reestablish your body to its normal state. Weiler Foundation is glad to be one of a handful of the offices in the country to offer you this progressive program.

Dr.Purissima M.Glaze

By the day's end, simply make certain to recollect that
beauty is health made noticeable!

Chapter 3

RELATING HEALTH TO BEAUTY

The association among Beauty and Health is instinctive. In some way or another, we as a whole comprehend that carrying on with a sound way of life works on our appearance, and that the strength of our skin is a mark of our general wellbeing. Yet, what a large number of us don't understand is that the association among Beauty and Health is similarly major areas of strength for as.

The Self-evident

Food, water, stress the executives, and rest are a higher priority than beauty care products and skincare items. Appropriately dealing with these four key fixings won't just make them look and feeling our best, yet in addition work on our wellbeing in manners we can't see. Presently, you most likely definitely know this, yet we should all's take a speedy boost prior to bouncing in to the not-really self-evident:

Food

Sugar, handled food varieties, refined starches, and even dairy all can cause irritation of our body's tissues. Breakouts in our skin are only one side effect of the horrendous idea of these substances in our bodies. They can frequently unleash devastation in our intestinal system and other body frameworks also.

The best arrangement is to eat all the more new entire food varieties, for example, products of the soil, particularly green vegetables that contain supplements and cell reinforcements that battle fundamental irritation.

Dr.Purissima M.Glaze

Water

This is maybe the clearest fixing to being our generally gorgeous. All things considered, our bodies are made out of somewhere near 60% water! Remaining hydrated permits supplements to all the more effectively arrive at our cells. It additionally lessens our skin's regular guard component - oil creation - which assists with clearing up our skin.

How much water would it be a good idea for us to drink? The Public Foundations of Sciences, Designing, and that's what medication verified, for individuals living in a mild climate, a satisfactory everyday liquid admission is around 15.5 cups (3.7 liters, or 125 oz) of water for men and around 11.5 cups (2.7 liters, or 91 oz) of water a day for ladies. That water can emerge out of various sources like juices and so forth, yet you're not getting it from diuretic beverages like sodas and espresso. Those beverages really dry out you, as a matter of fact. Thus, be cautious about what you go after in the refrigerator.

Stress The board and Exercise

At the point when we're focused on our endocrine framework discharges cortisol, a chemical that causes irritation, which can appear in our skin as skin break out, dermatitis, and different problems. Everybody oversees pressure in an unexpected way. Practice is one effective method for making it happen.

Routinely practicing works on our vascular framework and blood course which can increment cell turnover (supplanting of dead cells with new ones), and further develop complexion by conveying more oxygen to our cells.

Alternate ways of overseeing pressure include contemplation, yoga, strolling, and calm exercises, for example, perusing a book or simply investing some energy outside.

Rest

Rest allows our bodies an opportunity to mend. As per the Public Rest Establishment's rules, grown-ups ought to get somewhere in the range of seven and nine hours of rest each evening. What's more, only one evening of under seven hours of rest can increment dark circles, puffiness, and kinks.

The Not-Really Self-evident

In this way, we know being solid assists us with putting our best self forward. Be that as it may, think about what... putting our best self forward additionally assists us with being better. For reasons unknown, taking a couple of seconds to put on make-up, finish our hair and nails, or care for our skin may really add a long time to our lives.

Putting Our Best self forward = Living Better and Longer. At the point when we look great, we feel better. That is an easy decision. However, there's a developing group of logical proof that we're not simply feeling better since we look great; we really are better.

The mental experience of having a decent outlook on ourselves is known as emotional prosperity (SWB) and has been displayed to have huge long-and momentary medical advantages. At the point when we have SWB, we will quite often eat and rest better, go to specialists on a more regular basis, have expanded insusceptibility, and for the most part care more for ourselves.

Studies have demonstrated the way that SWB could expand our life span, amounting to seven and a half years to our lives. At the point when we deal with our skin, when we look our most gorgeous we upgrade our SWB, which thusly advances other taking care of oneself ways of behaving. After some time, this thought>action cycle prompts individual propensities that can affect our general prosperity. For instance, when we have an uplifting outlook, we will generally grin more, walk taller, have a sure step and visually engage. We set aside a few minutes for ourselves. We work out, scrub down, get manis and pedis, and subsequently, we feel and look more loose. More prominent certainty and unwinding energizes a positive identity, which builds up SWB.

Positive ways of behaving and perspectives likewise lead to additional wonderful relational encounters. Praises about how we look are called **certifiable input**. This supports our positive mental self view and the longing to keep on dealing with ourselves.

Chapter 4

OUR SKIN(BEAUTY) OUR HEALTH

Skin is one of the biggest organs of the body. Along these lines, really focusing on your skin can straightforwardly influence your general health/wellbeing. Your skin goes about as a defensive safeguard and is generally helpless against outside components. It's impacted by surprisingly factors. For example, the following can assume a part in your gene noral skin wellbeing:

- openness to UV radiation in tanning beds
- openness to substance poisons in tobacco
- unprotected sun openness for extensive stretches of time
- not getting sufficient rest, liquids, or sustenance
- maturing
- Dealing with your skin

There are steps you can take to guarantee you have sound skin. They incorporate the following:

- ➤ **Scrub**: Purge routinely, regularly two times day to day.
- ➤ Apply a toner subsequent to purifying in the event that you have slick skin.
- ➤ **Moisture**: Apply a lotion in the event that you have dry skin.
- ➤ **Exfoliate**: Peel to eliminate dead skin cells and light up your composition.

Other than an everyday skin health management schedule, practice it all the time to inspect your own skin for irregularities, stains, or some other changes consistently. Have your skin inspected by a specialist or dermatologist every year for any changes, or on the other hand if:

you have light complexion or numerous or huge moles

you are in the sun or use tanning beds

you have a past filled with skin issues, disturbances, or developments

It's additionally vital to shield your skin from a lot of endlessly sun harm, which might increment wrinkles as well as lead to skin disease. Cover your skin or use sunscreen to shield your skin from the harming beams of the sun. See your PCP or dermatologist assuming any skin disturbances or issues emerge.

Chapter 5

Understanding skin health management items

There are numerous items out there that are introduced as a dependable method for traveling back in time, for all time soften away cellulite, diminish kinks, and then some. Focus and investigate as needs be to conclude whether an item is truly vital for the soundness of your skin or on the other hand in the event that it's possibly destructive. Food and Medication Organization (FDATrusted Source) directs numerous items. It should direct items that change an individual's actual construction or biochemical cycles inside the body.

Items that are delegated beauty care products or dietary enhancements are not controlled. Instances of these include:

creams

hair shading

toothpaste

antiperspirant

nutrients

Your skin's surface is affected by outer components, similar to contamination and skin health management items, and inward components, including your wellbeing and diet. There are likewise normal changes that occur with age.

Wrinkles and other skin changes are important for life and nothing to be embarrassed about, yet assuming smooth skin is the thing you're pursuing, continue to peruse.

Here is our interaction.

Your skin's surface is impacted by outer components, similar to contamination and skin health management items, and inner components, including your wellbeing and diet. There are additionally normal changes that occur with age.

Wrinkles and other skin changes are important for life and nothing to be embarrassed about, however in the event that smooth skin is the thing you're pursuing, continue to peruse.

Chapter 6

Smooth skin schedule

Your way of life doesn't simply influence your general wellbeing. It influences your skin's wellbeing, as well. Here are a few solid living tips that can assist you with getting a charge out of smoother skin longer:

Remaining hydrated. However it's not completely clear precisely the way in which drinking water can work on your skin, there's evidenceTrusted Source that it does. Drinking water works on your skin's versatility and decreases indications of dryness and harshness, bringing about smoother skin.

Eating food varieties high in cell reinforcements. Cell reinforcement rich food varieties defensively affect the skin. These food varieties incorporate salad greens, yellow and orange products of the soil, and greasy fish, like salmon. There's likewise evidenceTrusted Source that adding probiotics to your eating regimen might help treat and forestall skin conditions, like dermatitis and skin break out, as well as skin harm brought about by bright (UV) light.

Working out. Creature and human studiesTrusted Source have demonstrated the way that standard vigorous activity can work on the skin's arrangement. It makes the skin's external layer more slender and thickens the internal layers — something contrary to what occurs as we age. This outcomes in smoother, more youthful looking skin.

Getting sufficient rest. Magnificence rest truly is a thing! Your skin, similar to the remainder of your body, fixes itself during rest. Expanded blood stream and collagen creation are several things that happen during rest and assist with fixing UV harm and lessen sun spots and kinks.

Safeguarding against the impacts of the sun. UV beams harm your skin cells' DNA, prompting untimely maturing, dryness, and a higher gamble of skin disease. Use sunscreen, limit your time in the sun, and wear defensive attire. Avoid tanning beds, which cause more harm than the sun, as indicated by the Food and Medication Organization (FDA)Trusted Source.

Not smoking. Interior and outer openness to tobacco smoke causes untimely skin maturing and wrinkles, and a higher gamble of skin problems, including skin inflammation and psoriasis. It additionally hinders your skin's capacity to mend itself. Stopping smoking can be troublesome, yet a specialist can assist with making a suspension plan that is ideal for you.

Drinking less liquor. Liquor utilization has been connected to skin photodamage, which is harm brought about by daylight. Drinking an excess of can likewise cause lack of hydration, which causes dry skin and untimely maturing. To diminish the impacts of liquor on your body and skin, limit your beverages to a couple each day.

Chapter 7

Solid skin items

There are various over-the-counter (OTC) items accessible to assist with keeping your skin smooth. Make certain to utilize items that are appropriate for your skin type for the best outcomes.

Skin exfoliators. Cleans can assist with sloughing ceaselessly dead skin cells that can develop on your skin, making it feel harsh and look lopsided. To peel securely, apply scour in a sluggish roundabout movement utilizing exceptionally light strain, and just shed one time each week.

Alpha hydroxy corrosive (AHA). AHAs are plant and creature acids utilized in healthy skin items. They peel, advance collagen and blood stream, and work on the presence of kinks. They're likewise used to treat skin inflammation and skin staining.

Creams. Cream adds an additional layer of security on your skin and assists it with remaining hydrated. Picking a facial lotion and applying it everyday can assist with keeping skin smooth. Remember to apply a saturating body salve to assist with keeping the remainder of your skin smooth.

Dry brushing. Dry brushing includes utilizing a characteristic, solid shuddered brush to peel the skin. Utilize the brush on dry skin, and brush in lengthy liquid strokes on your appendages, and in a roundabout movement on your back and middle.

Gentle, delicate cleaning agents. The American Foundation of Dermatology (AAD) suggests cleaning up with a delicate, nonabrasive, liquor free cleaning agent toward the beginning of the day and before bed, as well as in the wake of perspiring.

Chapter 8

Smooth skin home cures

Here are a few home cures that might further develop skin wellbeing for a smoother skin.

- Honey. Honey is a characteristic exfoliator that likewise ends up having bioactive properties that might be helpful in treating various skin conditions and lessening the presence of kinks.
- Coconut oil. Coconut oil is a powerful cream with mitigating and antimicrobial properties that might help likewise treat specific incendiary skin conditions. Since it might stop up pores, restricting its utilization to the body is ideal.
- Cereal showers. Cereal showers can assist your skin with holding dampness and treat specific skin conditions. You can make your own oats shower or shop for oats showers on the web, alongside other cereal healthy skin items for your face and body.

- Rejuvenating balms. A few rejuvenating balms, when weakened with transporter oils, can be applied to the skin to lessen kinks and treat various skin issues. A few medicinal balms for wrinkles incorporate lemon, rose, and jojoba oils.
- Humidifiers. Humidifiers add dampness to the air to keep your skin from drying out. It's likewise an impact solution for psoriasis. You can look for humidifiers on the web.

Chapter 9

Smooth skin medicines

Clinical medicines are accessible, contingent upon your requirements and spending plan. Address a dermatologist about your choices.

4% hydroquinone

Hydroquinone is a skin lightener that is utilized to treat hyperpigmentation. It can likewise be utilized to treat other skin issues, including:

skin break out scars

age spots

post-fiery imprints brought about by specific skin conditions

Compound strip

Compound strips eliminate dead skin cells so the better, smooth skin underneath is uncovered. It tends to be utilized to treat:

lopsided skin

almost negligible differences and kinks

scars

sun harm

melasma

Microdermabrasion and dermabrasion

Microdermabrasion utilizes an instrument with a grating tip to sand away the external layer of the skin. Dermabrasion is a more obtrusive technique that eliminates the harmed external layers of the skin.

Both can be utilized to treat:

almost irrelevant contrasts and wrinkles

hyperpigmentation,skin inflammation scars,clogged, pores, developed pores, lopsided complexion and surface

Laser skin reemerging

Laser skin reemerging utilizes strong light pillars to eliminate harmed skin. It very well may be utilized to lessen the presence of:

scars

stretch imprints

consume marks

age spots

Dermal fillers or Botox

Botox and dermal fillers are injectable restorative medicines utilized for wrinkles. Botox works by loosening up muscles in the face to streamline its appearance, while fillers utilize a gel-type substance to fill in lines and kinks. It likewise relax the forms of your face.

Chapter 10

Summary

In this chapter we try to put together virtually everything o Help you understand better.

Diet, exercise, and rest are three mainstays of a healthy life. The Connection Between Diet, Exercise, and Rest

Diet, exercise, and rest impact each other in complicated and endless ways.

Past actual health, beauty care products can assist with working on our mind-set, upgrade our appearance and lift our confidence. They can likewise assist with displaying individual style and, accordingly, are a significant method for social articulation.

Choosing the best beauty items for your skin type is a quality approach to working on your Health and appearance

Beauty Items implies skincare, individual consideration, scent, haircare and variety (beauty care products) items, for each situation including all parts, fixings, related devices and carries out thereof and apparatuses and embellishments for use in association therewith.

With what you should have gained from the Book you recently read, committing a skincare and Health errors will not be for you.